The Truth About the Eat Clean Diet

The Path to Health and Wellness

By: Miriam Welch

Publishers Notes

Disclaimer

This publication is intended to provide helpful and informative material. It is not intended to diagnose, treat, cure, or prevent any health problem or condition, nor is it intended to replace the advice of a physician. No action should be taken solely on the contents of this book. Always consult your physician or qualified health-care professional on any matters regarding your health and before adopting any suggestions in this book or drawing inferences from it.

The author and publisher specifically disclaim all responsibility for any liability, loss or risk, personal or otherwise, which is incurred as a consequence, directly or indirectly, from the use or application of any contents of this book.

Any and all product names referenced within this book are the trademarks of their respective owners. None of these owners have sponsored, authorized, endorsed, or approved this book.

Always read all information provided by the manufacturers' product labels before using their products. The author and publisher are not responsible for claims made by manufacturers.

Paperback Edition

Manufactured in the United States of America

DEDICATION

I dedicate this book to my parents who showed me how to be humble and to always help others, and also to my husband whose unfailing support has made me an even more confident person.

Table of Contents

Publishers Notes.......... 2

Dedication.......... 3

Table of Contents.......... 4

Chapter 1- What Is The Eat Clean Diet?.......... 5

Chapter 2- The Benefits Of The Eat Clean Diet.......... 9

Chapter 3- Who Is The Eat Clean Diet For?.......... 12

Chapter 4- Foods That Can Be Consumed On the Eat Clean Diet.......... 16

Chapter 5- How To Eat Clean When Away From Home.......... 22

Chapter 6- The Eat Clean Diet- Frequently Asked Questions.......... 26

Chapter 7- 10 Eat Clean Diet Recipes.......... 29

About The Author.......... 37

CHAPTER 1- WHAT IS THE EAT CLEAN DIET?

Eating clean is a lifestyle change that involves eating only the foods that would help you achieve a leaner, energetic, healthier you. No more junk or processed foods- only lean protein, good carbs and fats, fruits, veggies and water are allowed. In addition to exercising regularly, when on this diet, you can see a weight loss of around 3 pounds per week.

This diet was invented by Tosca Reno and includes a workout regime along with the approved list of foods. This diet isn't just about weight loss. Taking in less sugar and salt and staying away from processed "junk" foods lowers your cholesterol, makes your skin glow, and gives you longer lasting natural energy. The list goes on.

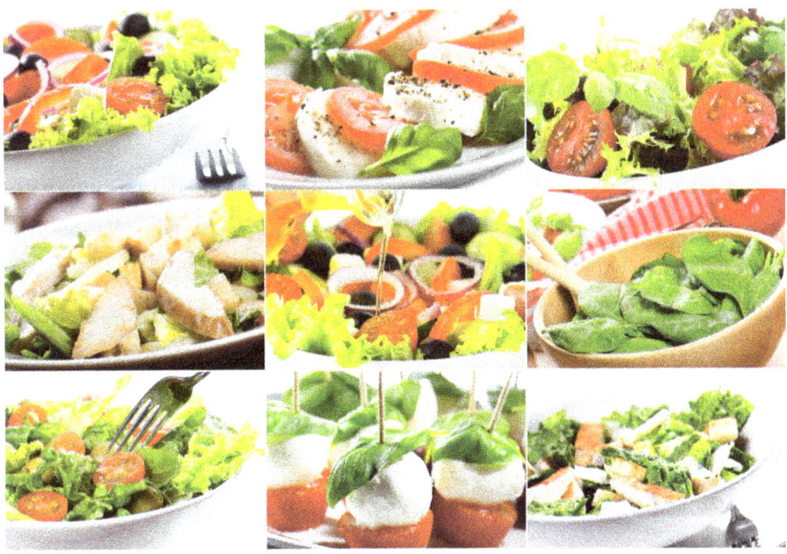

The eat clean diet is very well balanced. Your daily menu ensures that you have the proper serving of protein, fat, fruit, vegetables, and water daily. From the time you wake up to the time you go to sleep, you are actively engaging in certain aspects of your diet so that by the time the day is over, you will have taken in all the appropriate vitamins, nutrients, fiber, enzymes and energy that your body needs to function properly.

Most dieters often worry about feeling starved when they take on a diet challenge, but this diet will never leave you feeling hungry. For one, you have to consume an extra 4 to 6 cups of water on top of the normal 8 glasses that are required for daily consumption. Drinking a lot of water is filling without adding extra empty calories to your diet, while also providing your body with the essential vitamins and nutrients that you need.

Besides drinking lots of water, your meals are portioned so that you should be eating every 2 to 3 hours throughout the day, making a total of 6 meals. By eating several small meals in the day, the blood sugar stays at a constant level so that there should no longer be any sudden pangs of hunger or sudden food cravings.

Exercise is another important aspect of eating clean. Other diets will tell you that exercise is not necessary but this diet strongly encourages it. Exercise motivates you to keep doing your diet. It also gives you natural energy, a body in motion is far healthier than a sedentary body. The physical action of doing something is the motivator and long periods of inaction breeds laziness. Just eating right is only part of it and should be done in conjunction with staying active.

When on the eat clean diet, it is pretty strict as far as the types of things you should avoid. They include: processed foods, anything containing white flour and sugar, artificial sweeteners, sugary beverages, foods with preservatives or chemical additives, alcohol, artificial foods, anything with trans fats as well as any junk foods (chips, candy, crackers, cookies, etc.) as these are just empty calorie snacks with no nutritional values in them whatsoever.

So now that the things to avoid are out of the way, we can talk about what a typical day on this diet/lifestyle would entail. For starters, breakfast is an important meal of the day and should not be skipped. Within an hour of waking up in the morning, you should eat a simple breakfast. In two or three hours, your next small meal should be consumed. And every two to three hours thereafter, meals should be consumed, for a total of six meals per day. In between meals, you should be drinking plenty of water equaling around three to four liters for the day.

Check out recipe books for the perfect meals. Plan ahead and make sure your fridge and pantry are stocked so there is less temptation to stray from the plan. When shopping, only get items that have ingredients that you can pronounce and recognize. Stick to simple cooking with your meals containing 5 ingredients or less. It also helps to eat slower and listen to your body. Stop eating when you no longer feel hungry, as opposed to focusing on eating everything that is on your plate.

Tosca Reno offers great nutritional advice as well as meal plans. This one she used herself to lose a great amount of weight. The diet changed her life and she shares her secret so that those of us who want to lose weight and live healthier lives can do so too. Eating clean is incredibly popular because when you stick to it, it works! The fact that it works makes sense, considering sugar and salts, the very things that make us retain weight and damage the body are reduced significantly, if not eliminated altogether.

The hardest part of this plan (or any other), are to start it, to keep up with it for at least 30 days, and to stick to the do's and don'ts very carefully. People can be wary of being restricted to what they can and cannot eat and it can discourage someone easily. Rather than letting it discourage you, just put it into perspective: the things you are restricted from eating, are the very things you should not be eating in the first place! Rather than viewing the foods to avoid as restrictive, understand that they have no business entering your body at all. At least certainly not if you want to be healthy! Start Eating Clean and become a better you starting now!

Chapter 2- The Benefits Of The Eat Clean Diet

In the United States and abroad, many people have decided that they are going to start to implement the clean diet. The clean diet really is not a new concept; it is actually a concept that started in the 1960s. It was a time when people where deciding to try to eat whole foods that only came from the earth and foods that would give nutrition to their bodies and not just calories. Nowadays people are beginning to see the benefits of eating clean diet. Even though more Americans are going on diets; every year more people are diagnosed with diabetes, obesity, high cholesterol, high blood pressure, and heart disease. Many people now realize that they need to take their health back into their own hands and completely change the way that they are eating.

What It Means To Eat Clean

The concept of eating clean is very simple and basic. A person who is trying to eat on the clean diet is going to avoid any other food that has no nutritional value. Also important in the diet is to spread out meals over five or six small meals a day. Portion size is very important when it comes to the diet, and a person should eat meals that include whole grains, whole fruits, and whole vegetables. As mentioned in chapter 1, another part of the clean diet is to drink a lot of water, at least 8 cups a day. One should also avoid foods that are high in saturated fats and trans fats.

What Are The Benefits Of Eating Clean

The benefits of eating clean abound. The first thing that people will see when they begin to eat clean is that they will lose weight. There is generally a decrease in the amount of body fat from around 3 to 4 pounds per week. When a person is eating foods that only give nutrition to the body, their body will quickly respond and they will feel healthier. Apart from the physical aspects of eating healthy, there are other general improvements in a person's overall immunity. When a person's body is full of vitamins from healthy organic foods, they are able to maintain a higher immune system.

Diseases such as diabetes, stroke, cancers and heart attack all originate with a person's health. Even though a person cannot completely control if they will get a disease, when a person has a body that is healthy and an immune system that is functioning well, they will be less prone to disease.

Many people would find it interesting to know that by eating clean, they can also help their pocketbook. Eating Clean is actually a lot more cost-effective than people think. When a family goes out and eats fast food on a regular basis, or when they buy food that is prepackaged or frozen; they are going to be spending more money in the long run. When a family buys food that is whole, not only will they be eating food that is healthier, but their food will last them longer.

What To Expect When Eating Clean

There are some things that a person or family should expect when they decide that they are going to begin the new diet. The first thing, of course, that they should realize is that they are going to have to cook a lot more. It is simple to eat foods that are highly processed, because usually they can just go in the microwave or in the oven. When it comes to eating clean, a person has to actually cook their food completely, that may take more time; but the time is definitely worth it when a person realizes how many more nutrients he/she is giving to him/herself and family.

The next thing that a family or person has to realize when they decide to eat Clean is that they will have to pre-prepare their meals for lunch, and also if they are very busy in the evenings, they may have to do the same for dinner. The next thing that a person or family has to take into account when they are eating Clean is that some of their food may have to be flavored differently. A lot of unnatural flavors are very high in preservatives, additives, and chemicals. These have to be taken out of the clean diet and since that is the case, the family may have to find different herbs and seasonings for their food but with time they will enjoy the new flavors.

At first it may seem difficult for a family to eat Clean, but in reality, the basic concepts of eating Clean are very simple to get used to. When a family sees the benefits that eating clean gives to their health, it will make it even easier to change their lifestyle. Everyone realizes that we are all completely and totally in charge of what we eat each day. Therefore, it is up to us to decide how much of what we eat will affect our daily health in the long run. Even though it may be a lot easier to go out and eat food that is highly processed, it will have a negative impact on our health and there is no getting around that. Many families have made the smart choice to change their lives and change their diets. They have seen that eating Clean really gives them benefits, and they look and feel healthier and happier.

Chapter 3- Who Is The Eat Clean Diet For?

Have you ever considered taking steps toward an eat clean diet? Whether you want to fully adhere to the principles, or simply take baby steps toward the lifestyle, everyone can benefit from drinking plenty of water and mindfully eating a variety of wholesome foods. Read on for some strong reasons why there are a whole host of benefits associated with eating clean.

By drinking plenty of water, you keep your body hydrated and avoid habitually eating when you are actually just thirsty. Drinking enough water also helps to keep energy levels consistent and to ward off pesky dehydration headaches. Healthy water intake also assists with flushing toxins out of the body, and with absorbing important nutrients and vitamins. Sugary drinks such as sodas are void of nutrients, and even contain chemicals and sugars that contribute to gum disease and cavities. Oral health has an impact on overall health. Save your daily caloric intake for healthy foods, rather than empty nutrients that make your stomach bloated. Alcohol also has a lot of empty calories and can cloud judgment.

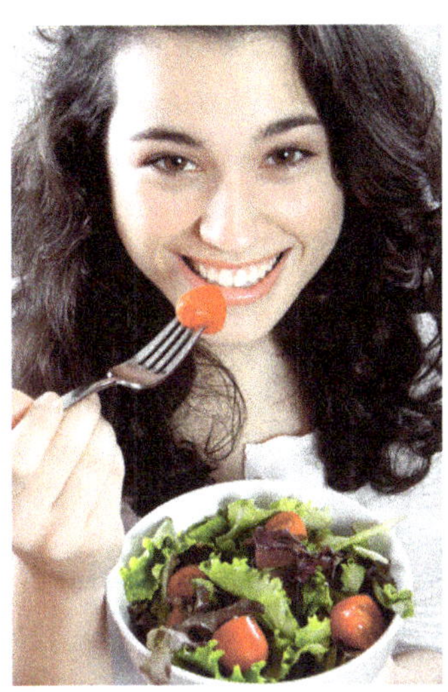

Everyone can experience clear judgment, optimal focus, and a burst of energy by starting the day by eating breakfast. People who skip breakfast often set themselves up for dietary failures before the day has even begun. The important thing is to not just eat breakfast, but eat a smart breakfast. Eat real, whole foods, and give yourself a great start to the day. Think breakfast items like eggs, oatmeal, and fresh fruit. Everyone from babies to the elderly does best by eating breakfast. If you have children living at home, be a good example for them and set them up for healthy eating habits.

Switching to whole foods rather than packaged foods also simplifies your life and cooking and eating habits. You will find yourself using fewer ingredients, and you will leave less of a footprint on the environment by eliminating unnecessary packaging. Most whole food remains can be composted and broken down.

Simplifying your snacks and meals doesn't mean creating boredom. Instead, eating whole foods slowly increases interest in your culinary experience. How wonderful to taste foods in their natural form and flavor! Take the time to truly taste and smell your food.

You will be satisfied with less, and perhaps even decrease your grocery bills, rather than increase them. Especially if you begin eating some meatless meals, you may notice a decrease in weekly or monthly grocery bills. You can still eat meat, just be sure that it is lean, and that you know where it came from. Look into purchasing meat straight from a butcher, rather than buying it prepackaged at a chain grocery store.

As you eat your small meals, take time to eat them slowly. Doing so allows you to become familiar with the feeling of being satisfied, rather than full. The brain takes a while to communicate a sense of fullness, so eating slowly allows the brain and digestive system the opportunity to be in sync.

If you are unfamiliar with where to purchase whole foods, consider joining a Community Supported Agriculture Program, or frequenting local farmer's markets. There are even grocery stores and natural food stores that feature organic produce and offerings such as freshly ground whole grain flours and nut butters. The fats found in nut butters are acceptable on an eating clean diet because it is the kind of fat that is actually good for your heart.

By avoiding processed foods, you will also avoid preservatives and artificial sweeteners. Although there may be a period of adjustment, your taste buds will begin to crave the tastes and textures of the whole foods that you are eating. You will experience improvements in your overall health, without counting calories or learning complicated diets or lifestyle plans.

As you make the switch to eating clean, be aware of hidden sugars and preservatives in foods that you may currently consider to be healthy. Read labels and kick the sugar habit. As you eliminate sugar, you will be pleasantly surprised to find yourself craving it less and less. The same principle works with a variety of unhealthy fats. Chemical additives can be addictive, but you can train your body to have affections for healthier kinds of foods.

Eating frequent small meals also keeps your metabolism going and helps to prevent binge eating. Really be aware of portion sizes. It is hard to see progress when you are eating too much food, whether it is healthy or not.

If you plan to incorporate any vitamins or supplements in your diet, you need to consult your physician first. While physicians across the board agree eating whole foods helps support mental health and ward off disease, caution and consideration need to be used when introducing vitamins and supplements into the mix.

If you feel unstable about sticking with an eating clean diet, take time and map out a weekly meal plan. Remember to account for a variety of small meals daily. Think ahead about what you will include in these small meals. You may even want to post this information in a prominent place in the kitchen where you or everyone in your family can easily see it and access it.

Incorporating clean eating is good for everyone, young and old. It doesn't need to be overwhelming, and you can gradually work toward achieving the total lifestyle. Be gracious, and give yourself time to adjust to clean eating. Chances are, you will love the results! Continue to the next chapter to learn what foods can be included in the eat clean diet.

Chapter 4- Foods That Can Be Consumed On the Eat Clean Diet

Why should you eat clean? Eating a whole food, unprocessed diet enables you to have more energy, it encourages a healthy weight, and it improves your overall health. Unfortunately, most of us have spent our entire lives eating the processed foods that are so prevalent in the standard American diet. This prompts many of us to throw our hands up in the air and exclaim "What do I eat?"

Eating clean is one of the easiest things you can do to improve your health, and it's easy too. Simply eat unprocessed foods in their natural state. A great example would be to opt for a real piece of fruit to snack on, instead of a processed fruit roll-up. Trust me; fruit tastes so much better than the processed versions. To make things easier, I am going to list the many foods you can enjoy, while on this diet.

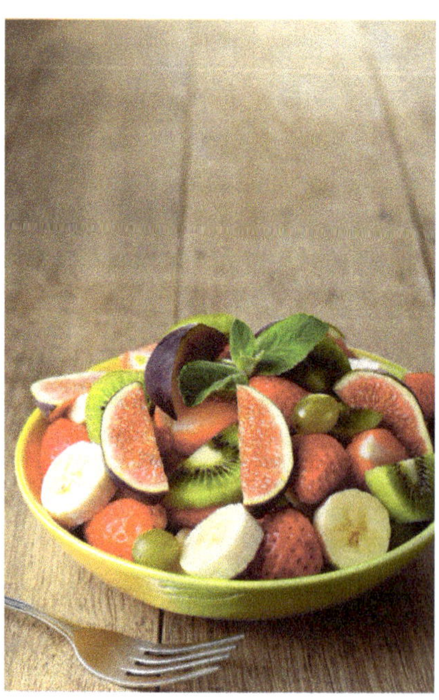

Vegetables

Leafy greens are the superstars of this group; vegetables such as Kale, Collard Greens, Romaine Lettuce, and many more. Vegetables have many health benefits. They are loaded with Vitamins A, C, E, and K. They are also rich in Minerals, like Calcium, Iron, and Potassium. There is also an abundance of Antioxidants and Phytonutrients, both of which have outstanding benefits to health and longevity. Here is a list of some of the better known ones.

- Kale
- Collard Greens
- Kohlrabi
- Bok Choy
- Carrots
- Potatoes
- Chard
- Artichokes
- Spinach
- Sweet Potatoes
- Parsnips
- Rutabaga
- Mustard Greens
- Romaine Lettuce
- Beets
- Avocados
- Asparagus
- Bell Peppers
- Cauliflower
- Broccoli
- Cauliflower
- Mushrooms
- Celery
- Cabbage
- Eggplant
- Fennel
- Green Beans
- Garlic
- Beet Greens
- Onions
- Green Peas
- Summer Squash
- Winter Squash
- Tomatoes
- Turnip Greens
- Leeks
- Corn
- Cucumbers
- Celeriac

Fruits

Fruits and Berries are wonderful sources of many valuable nutrients. These tasty treats are loaded with Vitamins C, A, E, the B

Vitamins, and Vitamin K. They are also rich in several minerals, such as Potassium, and Magnesium. Fruits, like vegetables, are also rich in Antioxidants, and Polyphenols. It is recommended that you have at least 9 servings of fruits and vegetables every day. So Instead of having cake for desert, why not have a fruit salad? Here are some tasty fruits:

- Apples
- Pears
- Oranges
- Grapefruit
- Lemons
- Persimmons
- Mango
- Papaya
- Kiwi
- Nectarines
- Figs
- Dates
- Strawberries
- Raspberries
- Cantaloupe
- Bananas
- Blackberries
- Pineapples
- Plums
- Prunes
- Grapes
- Watermelon
- Apricots

Beans and Legumes

Rich in vegetarian protein, Beans and Legumes are an important addition to a clean, healthy diet. They offer a myriad of health benefits, such as lowering cholesterol, reducing the risk for coronary artery disease, lowering blood pressure, and stabilizing blood sugars. They are also an important aid in weight control. Beans and Legumes are fiber rich. When you eat them, you feel satisfied longer. So by feeling full, you reduce your food intake without increasing hunger. Instead of a cheeseburger, try a bean burger on a whole grain bun. You will love it.

- Black beans
- Dried peas
- Garbanzo beans
- Kidney beans
- Lentils
- Lima beans

- Pinto beans
- Cranberry beans
- Soy beans
- Peas
- Fava beans
- Navy beans
- Northern beans
- Red beans

Lean Protein

Protein is essential to a healthy diet. Let your protein sources be as lean and healthy as possible. Protein improves the health of your cardiovascular system, and is a must for healthy hair, skin, and nails. Another plus for lean protein: They help to stabilize weight too! There are animal sources, and an abundance of vegetarian sources. Here are some of your options:

- Tofu
- Lean Chicken Breast
- Lean cuts of Turkey
- Tempeh
- Beans
- Eggs
- Lean Beef
- Seafood

Healthy Fats

For many years the nutritional establishment told us that fat was bad. Think again. Research has shown that healthy, whole food forms of fat are essential to a clean, health supportive diet. They have been discovered to have many benefits, both mentally and physically. Healthy fats have been shown to strengthen your immune system. Fats from whole foods have also been shown to help with heart disease, diabetes, and weight control. The trick to enjoying these good fats is to get the majority of them from whole food sources, like nuts, seeds, avocados and fish. Use free flowing oils sparingly. Here are some excellent sources of healthy fats.

- Avocados
- Peanuts
- Cashews
- Flax seeds
- Chia Seeds
- Olives

- Macadamia nuts
- Brazil nuts
- Soy products
- Olive oil
- Avocado oil
- Hazelnut oil
- Salmon
- Walnuts Pecans
- Sesame seeds
- Spices

Fresh Spices not only make your food taste delicious, they are incredibly good for you too. Certain spices may protect your health in many ways. They help prevent cancers, coronary artery disease, high blood pressure, and diabetes. They are also a delicious way to help kick start your immune system! Many of our common herbal remedies are derived from them. Spices are also known to be nutritional power houses. Many commonly used spices are rich in Vitamins, Minerals, and Antioxidants. When using them, fresh is best. Powdered versions can be good, but fresh garlic trumps the powdered kind any day. You never knew that good health could be so spicy!

- Basil
- Black Pepper
- Cayenne Pepper
- Chili Pepper
- Cilantro
- Cinnamon
- Cloves
- Cumin
- Dill
- Ginger
- Mustard Seeds
- Oregano
- Parsley
- Peppermint
- Rosemary
- Thyme
- Turmeric
- Garlic

At first, eating a clean, whole foods diet might seem like a challenge but as you learn and discover more about it, you discover that not only does eating this way benefit you nutritionally, it does so in many other ways, physically, mentally, as well as in the way you interact with your environment. Whole foods contribute to a more holistic you. The journey is worth it.

Chapter 5- How To Eat Clean When Away From Home

With clean eating gaining, if not in popularity, then certainly in awareness, it's becoming easier than ever to eat healthy away from home. This is real life, after all, so no one needs to be chained to the kitchen and local greengrocer to maintain a diet of whole, unprocessed foods. Healthy alternatives are everywhere. All it takes is some forethought so decisions are easy and choices are abundant.

Remember that the same rules apply away from home as they do in a structured environment. Stay mindful of the point of clean eating, which is to eat whole foods prepared without chemicals or preservatives. There are a myriad of options for sticking with a healthy lifestyle choice of eating a clean diet. Here are suggestions to help you make wise, guilt-free decisions while away from home:

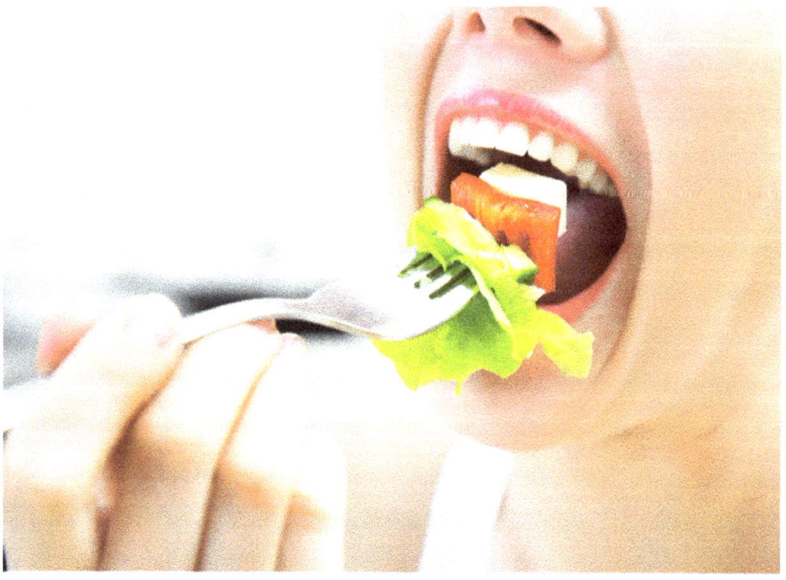

If being away for the day, perhaps while at work is in question, the answer is easy. Pack meals and snacks from home. Buy one of the many styles of coolers that looks like a handbag, and fill it with foods from the refrigerator. Salads, hard boiled eggs, fruits, homemade crust-less veggie quiches and soups are all easy to eat in an office lunch-time environment. Snacks can include:

- An organic yogurt,
- An apple or banana with a tablespoon of all-natural peanut butter
- A handful of nuts with dried fruit
- An all-natural applesauce cup
- Crudités with hummus or guacamole
- A cup of sliced berries

Some of those same options work well to carry when traveling. Who really wants to eat airplane food, anyway? Skip the 100-year-old bag of goldfish and pack snacks from home. TSA won't do a strip-search for carrying an apple on board, so tuck one in a carry-on bag. There are even several brands of all-natural bars that can be kept in a handbag for long periods of time.

Of course eating in restaurants is not only unavoidable; it's one of life's pleasures and should be embraced accordingly. Again, prepare in advance so that socializing doesn't include veering off the path of clean eating. When at all possible, take responsibility for choosing the restaurant. Seafood and sushi restaurants are easy options, as are vegan establishments.

Meet friends for lunch rather than dinner, where meals are usually lighter and there are often several clean choices readily available. There is also less pressure to drink, which may weaken your resolve. Even then, keep reading because there are solutions for social drinking, too.

Regardless of the restaurant, eat something from home prior to going out. Have some protein and a bit of whole grain to satisfy hunger and keep the temptation of the bread basket or dessert cart at bay. It's no secret that sourdough and cheesecake are not your friends, but chicken breast and veggies will love you forever. Show your clean and healthy friends the love right back!

Check out restaurant menus online prior to dining out. Select a clean meal beforehand so looking at the specials or hearing what friends are ordering isn't an issue.

Drink plenty of water both before going out and while dining. Filling up on water is another way to quell the urge to pick at foods that are less than optimum choices.

Don't even look at the Fettuccine Alfredo across the table! Make a commitment to stick to the plan knowing that the lean, clean feeling will far outweigh a weak moment with cream-laden complex carbs.

Even if an occasion rises when there is no time to prepare or anticipate eating away from home, you can still anticipate what isn't immediately in your control. Ask to have foods prepared without sauces. Ask to have your dish steamed or at least made with olive oil. Stick with the simplest dishes such as:

- Grilled, steamed or raw fish
- Grilled meats,
- Steamed or sautéed veggies
- A naked sweet potato

These are foods that will fill you up and allow you to enjoy dining out without compromising a clean eating program.

Yes, and then there is the question: to drink or not to drink? The short answer is, "not if you can help it". The longer answer is that sometimes having a drink is appropriate and other times, well, who doesn't want to lift a glass with friends or loved ones? In this case, too, there are intelligent ways to imbibe. Say no to the bubbly. The sugar content is ghastly. The same is true for fruity or creamy mixes, most of which are canned and made with preservatives. Want a cocktail? Opt for gin or vodka, which are the least processed liquors. Try mixing with club soda and a splash of fresh squeezed grapefruit juice or big twist of lemon. The fizz of the soda feels festive and, because you've 'picked your poison', no bartender will try to persuade you to do shots of Goldschläger to liven up! If limited to beer and wine, go for white wine mixed with club soda. The sugar in the wine is cut by adding club soda. Drinking the extra soda water never hurts, either.

With so many choices available, it's possible to enjoy a full and happy social and professional life that includes eating away from home and dining out in restaurants. Step out armed with a plan and the determination to stay on course for what is making you look and feel fabulous by eating clean every day.

Chapter 6- The Eat Clean Diet- Frequently Asked Questions

What is the Eat Clean diet?

The Eat Clean diet was created by nutritionist and health enthusiast, Tosca Reno. Reno debuts her newest book as the Renovation of diet and self. Based on maintaining a clean and healthy lifestyle, this diet targets only clean foods that are not processed. The diet promotes only eating natural foods to increase health and vitality. It is not just about losing weight but about building a healthy core from the inside out. It helps you to identify bad eating habits and sets a course for changing these habits and the ability to appreciate real foods.

With the busy lives many of us lead and the battle to live a safe healthy lifestyle, eating clean may seem like a hassle. But, with Reno's guidance, making the switch from fast foods and junk to a healthy diet is easy. Eating healthy foods and building healthy life goals is easy to obtain when you set the proper patterns. Breaking free of bad habits can be obtained when given the proper blueprint to follow and the diet is much more than healthy recipes and diet tips but also a map for a healthier lifestyle

Tosca also has delivered her new book with a very personable air and travels the road of trying to gain a healthier core. She highlights her own battles of identifying healthy foods and supplementing them into her busy lifestyle. She embarks the readers upon the future of what we need to eat to turn around the very real health crisis that unhealthy foods have caused and gives the readers hope, guiding her readers to make these very necessary changes.

Are There Recipes in the Eat Clean diet Book?

Yes. The book is full of healthy recipes that target a healthy diet regimen. These recipes will help in identifying the best foods for eating clean and how to make healthy meals the entire family will love. Sometimes it seems impossible to include the whole family in healthy eating but the information Reno has provided helps to include implementing the entire family equally. Recipes will vary from lavish dinners to easy-to-make snacks that adults and children will love. You will find useful recipes in the next chapter.

Can You Lose Weight on the Eat Clean diet?

The diet is not geared to create fast weight loss. The problems with diets that promote fast weight loss is that they do not target the health of the body but the starvation techniques of weight loss, and often the results do not last. When following this diet, you can experience weight loss on an average of three pounds a week and these are pounds you will lose for good. The diet is targeted to build a healthy balance between life and food and will help those who need to lose weight and those who may need to gain weight.

The safest way to lose weight is naturally and without gimmicks or starving your body of necessary food groups. Eating only meat for weeks may help to jump start a weight loss plan but is not a lifelong practice that promotes health. The Eat Clean diet will help with weight loss but does not exclude any food groups or use crazy meal plans. The idea is to purify the diet and the body as a whole improving health and impressing the body to maintain a healthy weight.

Are the Recipes Easy to Use?

The foods in the eat clean diet are natural and normal fresh foods that are available everywhere. The recipes are created for simplicity and ease. There are also provided shopping lists that help you to plan and follow a clean diet menu. Reno has attacked every area of learning to eat healthy and has provided the best instruction possible. Making such large diet changes can not only be a hassle but also become overwhelming, the Eat Clean diet will help with the changes and guide you through the necessary steps. The recipes are easy to follow and the shopping lists help to break down the recipes while following what's in season and the best foods to buy or substitute when necessary.

Is It Affordable?

One of the major problems with diets is that the recipes are great but use some very expensive foods. The Eat Clean diet does not use overly fancy recipes and everyone can afford to fit the new meal plans into their budget. If you are a family who may eat out a lot, you may even notice that you are not only eating better but saving a lot of money as well.

This diet is a breakthrough to healthy living and creating lifelong eating habits that can improve the lifestyle of the entire family. You can learn to improve your health and target main issues such as weight, diabetes, lethargy and illness. Learning to eat healthy and remove all fake foods and foods that cause unhealthy issues is the first in the line of defenses against the many things that can bring us down. Having more life and energy and living with vitality is the boost we all need and this diet delivers.

Chapter 7- 10 Eat Clean Diet Recipes

As we have seen throughout this book, clean eating and dieting has become the preferred method for those seeking to rid their bodies of toxins and eat in a much simpler and cleaner manner that facilitates better total body well-being. These ten great clean diet recipes range from breakfast to dinner and even include some great snacks.

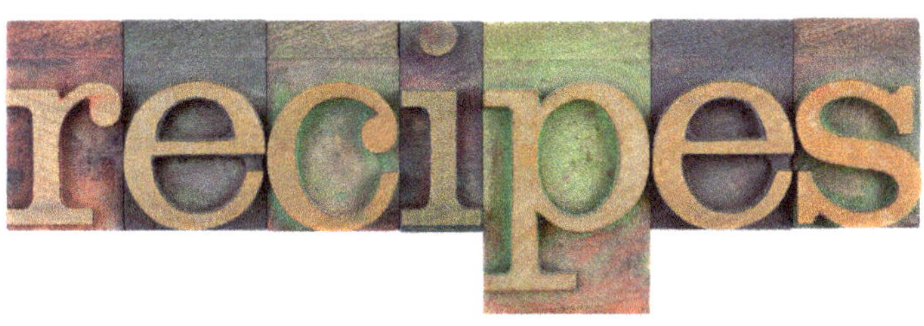

Carrot Ginger Soup

Ingredients:

- 1 to 2 tablespoons of sesame or olive oil
- 3 or 4 shallots finely minced
- 1 pound of organic carrots, peeled and diced
- 1 cup of vegetable stock, low or reduced sodium
- 1 cup Greek style plain yogurt
- 1 Bunch of fresh mint

Instructions:

- Sauté the shallots in the oil until translucent. Set aside.

- Boil the carrots in the vegetable stock until the carrots are fork tender.
- Cool the carrots and keep in the broth.
- Puree the carrots in a blender until smooth.
- Add the shallots and blend once more to make the soup creamy.
- Top the soup with Greek yogurt and a few sprigs of fresh mint.

Crabby Eggs

Ingredients:

- 1 dozen cage free brown eggs
- 1 pound fresh lump crab meat
- 1 cup Greek yogurt, plain
- 1 teaspoon seafood seasoning, low sodium
- 1 teaspoon minced shallots or garlic
- 1/4 teaspoon yellow mustard

Instructions:

- Place eggs in a pot of cold water, covering the eggs with water and bring to a rolling boil.
- Turn off the heat and cover the eggs with a lid. Let the eggs sit for 20 minutes.
- Peel the eggs and cut in half lengthwise.
- Remove the yolk and place in a bowl.
- Add to the yolk all remaining ingredients and whisk until smooth.
- Fill the eggs with the crab mixture for a great midday snack.

Parmesan Potatoes

Ingredients:

- 1 pound potatoes, organic, cleaned and cut in to strips
- 1 to 2 tablespoons extra virgin olive oil
- 1 teaspoon onion powder
- 1 teaspoon garlic powder
- 1 teaspoon oregano
- 1/2 cup grated Parmesan cheese

Instructions:

- Place oil on a baking sheet and coat the entire sheet.
- Place the potato strips on the sheet in a single layer.
- Sprinkle all spices evenly over the potatoes and bake for 30 minutes at 425 °F or until crisp.
- Flip the potatoes once, halfway through the baking process.
- Remove from the oven, place in a bowl and toss with the Parmesan cheese.

Deconstructed Egg Sandwich

Ingredients:

- 2 cage free brown eggs
- 1 tablespoon olive or sesame oil
- 1 thick slice of fresh avocado
- 1 thick slice of tomato
- Fresh cilantro
- Sea salt to taste
- Red pepper flakes (to taste)

Instructions:

- Prepare the egg by heating the oil in a pan and then breaking the eggs right in to the pan so the yolk is facing up.
- Cook for 3 to 5 minutes until the edges are bubbling and the yolk has solidified.
- Place the egg, yolk side up on a plate and top with the avocado, tomato, a pinch of salt (to taste), red pepper flakes for a little heat and a sprig of fresh cilantro.

Hot Potato Chips

Ingredients:

- 1 pound baby potatoes cut into small circles
- 2 lemons
- 2 tablespoons olive oil
- Sea salt and fresh black pepper

Instructions:

- Toss the potatoes in the olive oil to coat all pieces.
- Grate the zest of one lemon into the bowl, and juice both lemons into the bowl as well: toss again.
- Place the potatoes on a baking sheet and bake at 450 °F for 30 minutes or until crisp and brown.
- Serve hot and crispy as a snack or side dish twist.

Lime Shrimp

Ingredients:

- 2 pounds raw, de-veined fresh or frozen shrimp
- 2 to 3 garlic cloves minced fine
- 2 to 3 limes
- Sea salt and fresh black pepper to taste
- Olive oil

Instructions:

- Place the olive oil in a sauté pan so that there is a good one inch in the pan.
- Heat the oil.
- While the oil is heating place shrimp in a bowl and toss with the minced garlic and the zest and juice of the limes.
- Season (to taste) with salt and pepper and place shrimp in the hot oil.
- Sauté until the shrimp curls and turns pink. Top with cilantro and serve warm.

Breakfast Smoothies

Ingredients:

- 1 apple, peeled, cored and diced
- 1 carrot peeled and diced
- 3 leaves fresh spinach, washed, dried and chopped
- 1 banana cubed
- 1 teaspoon vanilla extract
- 1 cup Greek yogurt
- 1 cup almond milk

Instructions:

- Place all fruits and vegetables in a blender with the vanilla and almond milk.
- Puree until smooth.
- Add the Greek yogurt and pulse to blend well.
- Serve cold and right away.

Open Face Quesadilla

Ingredients:

- 6 whole wheat and gluten free tortillas
- 1 pound white meat chicken, cooked and sliced in thin strips
- 1 avocado cut into thin strips
- 1 small red onion sliced thin
- 1 cup goat cheese
- 1 cup fresh salsa
- 1/2 cup Greek yogurt
- Salt, pepper and cilantro for garnish and flavor

Instructions:

- Place one tortilla on a plate, cover with a damp paper towel, place another on top and repeat the process until all six are on the plate and the stack is topped with one last damp towel.
- Microwave for one minute to heat.
- Place a heated tortilla on a plate and top with chicken, avocado, onion, cheese, salsa and yogurt.
- Garnish with cilantro and salt and pepper to taste.

Chickpea Pops

Ingredients:

- 2 cups chickpeas, cooked and drained
- 1 tablespoon each garlic powder, onion powder, oregano, red pepper flakes and cumin
- 1 to 2 tablespoons olive oil

Instructions:

- Toss the chickpeas in a bowl with all ingredients until well coated.
- Spread out evenly on a baking sheet and roast at 350 °F for 30 to 45 minutes or until crunchy.
- Serve warm or room temperature as a snack.

Clean Buffalo Chicken

Ingredients:

- 1 pound cage free chicken breast, sliced thin
- 1 cup Panko
- 1 cup Greek yogurt
- 1/4 to 1/2 cup Buffalo chicken wing hot sauce
- 1 egg, beaten

Instructions:

- Preheat oven to 375 °F.
- Whisk together the egg and yogurt until smooth.
- Dip a slice of chicken in the egg and yogurt mixture and then coat with Panko.
- Place on oil-coated baking sheet.

- Repeat until all chicken has been breaded.
- Bake for 30 minutes or until crisp and cooked thoroughly.
- Remove from oven and drizzle the hot sauce on top of the chicken strips.

About The Author

Miriam Welch has always been careful about what she eats. She grew up in a family of extremely healthy eaters and this is something that she never forgot. She has written quite a number of books, but the one topic that she loves to write about is the clean diet.

Miriam knows what it is to eat clean and merely wants to help her readers to learn the basics of a way of eating that our ancestors used to follow centuries ago. Eating clean requires the individual to refrain from eating junk foods and other processed foods.

www.ingramcontent.com/pod-product-compliance
Ingram Content Group UK Ltd.
Pitfield, Milton Keynes, MK11 3LW, UK
UKHW021828270726
14058UKWH00001B/44

9 781680 329322